Caring for
Your Health
and
My Thoughts
on
God's Role

David Ilo, MD

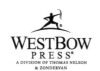

WESTBOW
P R E S S®
A DIVISION OF THOMAS NELSON
& ZONDERVAN

WestBow Press books may be ordered through booksellers or by contacting:

WestBow Press
A Division of Thomas Nelson & Zondervan
1663 Liberty Drive
Bloomington, IN 47403
www.westbowpress.com
1 (866) 928-1240

ISBN: 978-1-5127-6177-1 (sc)
ISBN: 978-1-5127-6178-8 (e)

Library of Congress Control Number: 2016917805

Print information available on the last page.

WestBow Press rev. date: 10/27/2016

This book is dedicated to my special mentor and dad Dr Matthias O Ilo (RIP), my mum Grace Ilo, my wife Piper Smith Ilo and all my siblings including Joel C Ilo, Esther U Ilo (RIP), Winifred C Ilo, Judith O Ilo, Euphemia O Ilo and Lidia I Ilo.

My dedication is also, to the doctors and the nurses that work with me in the hospitals, nursing homes and hospice.

I will reserve special praise to my patients who have taught me more than the care I give them. May God continue to Bless all of them and give them hope even at the most difficult times. May God give me grace to care for them like I would care for my own. May I continue to have in my mind (all the time), that anyone created by God could be a patient. And that those patients deserve to be treated with utmost dignity.

Contents

Introduction

This book is a way of expressing myself in what I have learned as a physician, starting when I was a child up to the present. I've always been very good with observation; as a physician, observation is the key to success. My specialty includes internal medicine and age management medicine, and I do a lot of work with patient rehabilitation. I'm also a hospice physician in Fort Wayne, Indiana, with a lot of experience as a hospitalist physician (a physician who specializes in acute care). I also manage the elderly in nursing homes and hospitals. I'm a Catholic and a strong believer in Jesus Christ. I'm also a strong believer in miracles after doing independent research on the topic.

I believe that we have a role in our health care, though I still believe that God's role is there too, just like with the issues of miracles. I also believe we encounter miracles every day, though we may not take it seriously. For example, we might have been in a big accident, but we survived it without a scratch—we might not even know how we survived it.

For the most part, however, we are responsible for our own health care. I see the role of God in destiny as occasional, and it happens less frequently than some of us believe. I see some people who have taken very good care of themselves, especially in developed countries, and they are better off than those who have not. Those in wealthy countries do better, health-wise, than the poor countries. We also see that death is everywhere and that there seems to be a balance, which shows that the Almighty is watching us.

I believe most of us are given a fair chance to live a healthy life. I also believe that life in Christ helps us to understand life better. Sometimes we live our lives not just for ourselves but also to help people around us. I believe that there are ways we touch other people's lives because of our strong Christian beliefs.

Atheists may not believe in God, but my biggest influence in writing this book was from the wife of an atheist who had a colon cancer and who was in her eighties.

She told me to write this book to encourage people, not just as a health care worker but to help a lot of people with spiritual richness. I learned from her that the greatest strength she had was born from her total belief in God. Her message was that it is left to the spirit to fight when you are down.

This book will mostly be about caring for our health and how to prevent common diseases and live longer. I'll demonstrate God's influence with a story my dad told me. This type of story doesn't happen every day, but, like miracles, it happens so the world will know that God exists. Such stories have been described as paranormal, but this doesn't change the fact that God has given us authority over most things, including our health.

My dad's story is unique because he was an educated man and a strong believer in science. My dad was born in Nigeria but moved to England to study as a teenager and lived there for a long time. He was lonely in England, however, and always was thinking about his brothers and sisters back home. He felt so isolated that when he returned to Nigeria in the seventies with my mum, my brother, and me, he swore he would never go back to England.

One memorable aspect about my dad's stay in England was his mum's apparition at bedtime. My grandmother was dead, but this vision didn't stop until a certain thing happened—that's the twist of the story.

The United Kingdom had just granted Nigeria the power to rule itself. At that time, anyone with a sponsor could immigrate to England and become a citizen. My dad took advantage of this opportunity to study engineering.

His desire to go back to Nigeria was even more intense after a civil war that involved the Nigerian and Biafran armies. Biafra lost the war, and infrastructures were destroyed and many lives lost.

My dad was pro-Biafra; he had a beard and mustache similar to that of the Biafran leader. To him, going back to Nigeria was a must.

While in England, my dad saw his mum sitting close to him whenever he was about to turn in for the night. Usually, this vision of his mum would tell my dad everything that was going on with his ten brothers in Nigeria. She would give my dad all of the details about the war and how his family had survived one attack or another. As a scientist, my dad didn't believe in ghosts, but he would speak to the apparition, saying, "Okay, thank you for telling me." My dad felt it must have been a dream, but whenever he communicated with his family, he learned that everything was as the vision had told him.

The most important thing is that my dad started to believe the "dreams" were real. So he started asking questions of the vision, and she either would answer them or pretend not to hear them.

One question she would never answer was whether she was dead. According to my dad, he put the question to the vision to see her reaction, which was always the same: she would change the topic and talk about something else.

At some point, my dad started thinking that he might not be asleep but awake. However, the vision would talk to him until he fell into a deep sleep. The fact that this happened most nights actually prevented my dad from feeling lonely any longer.

It should be noted that my grandmother died during that war, and the news was sent to my dad via telegram. Yet this vision was in my dad's house most nights while he was living by himself in England. The vision was recurring until my dad married my mum. My grandmother told my dad that she had good news for him.

"What good news?" my dad asked.

She said, "Well, your senior brother found a wife for you today, and her name is Grace. She is beautiful, and I would like you to marry this girl." She then gave my dad a description of the girl. This was part of an arranged marriage, which is still common in Nigeria.

At that time, to make a phone call from Nigeria to England, you had to travel many miles to get to a central line. When my uncle called my dad to tell him about his search for a wife, my dad asked him if her name was Grace.

My uncle was surprised when my dad told him the name, but he said, "Yes, her name is Grace. How did you know?"

My dad didn't know how to tell him the story, as he was embarrassed to even say it. He decided that he would tell his brother at the right time.

My dad was almost sure the vision was real, but he still had some doubt because it defied science, and he was a scientist. He had been a good Catholic and an altar boy. All along in his church teachings, the priest had told my father there was no such thing as ghosts, though a vision could be a better explanation.

However, my dad's explanation of the event was that this could be a dream. For me, his explanation was too simple, but my dad was a smart man. He did everything necessary for the marriage to take place. The two families agreed on a traditional marriage, and after that, my mum had to join my dad in England, where they would have a Christian marriage.

On the night when she boarded the plane to England, the vision appeared before my dad as usual, when he was about to go to sleep. My grandmother told my dad that she was nervous and didn't want my dad to miss my mum when she arrived. During those times, when communication was poor and airports and airplanes were few, it was possible to lose a friend or a fiancé when they arrived from another country.

She described my mum again and what she was wearing. My dad took note of the description that night without even thinking twice. At that time, my dad was almost 100 percent sure of the correct prediction of this "dream."

As my dad waited in the airport, he thought of the description the vision had given him, which included the color of my mum's clothing. When he saw a woman who matched the description, he called out, "Grace?"

My mum turned and said, "Yes. Are you Mathias?"

My dad replied in the affirmative.

They had never seen each other before that day. Usually in an arranged marriage, there's a protocol the couple must follow to see each other, but my dad decided to breach the protocol. My mum was nervous, as it was her first time in England and the first time she had traveled outside Nigeria. She also was surprised that my dad had called her by name. "How did you know it was me?" she asked.

My dad said, "I had your description and what you were wearing."

"How did you get that?" she asked.

My dad said, "I'll let you know after we get home."

When they got there, my dad explained about the vision. "Sometimes it looks so real," he said, "but I feel the vision is a kind of paranormal communication because I have no friends and have been lonely."

Loneliness is the biggest challenge that immigrants face in a new country. Most of their friends are in their home country, and then there's also the culture shock. Most immigrants compensate by working harder and occasionally looking for people from their country of origin in the new country. In the sixties and seventies, there were few people from Ibo and Nigeria in England, so my dad felt alone. At that time—sometimes even now—it was difficult to find friends, even if you tried. Part of the reason was the culture shock, but it was even worse if you were proud about your beliefs. It also was worse if the immigrant was ethnocentric and believed everyone was like him or her.

As they say, we always see the worst of us in others. My perspective, as a physician and someone who deals with the elderly and dying people, is that God works in mysterious ways, and there are things we cannot yet explain.

Stories like this one may be the only ones

available to us, but this doesn't change the fact that we have to do our own part to improve our lives. We shouldn't be discouraged by the slight misfortune that could happen. We should see the good result of those who have worked hard to be where they are. We shouldn't dismiss people's success as just luck; we should try to see if there's anything we could learn from them.

Believing in destiny isn't bad, but, like miracles, I believe it's not what defines us. I also know that Jesus raised Lazarus from the dead, but Lazarus still died. I believe Jesus raised Lazarus to prove that Jesus was the Resurrection.

Jesus didn't go around Jerusalem raising all the dead people. He performed occasional miracles to show his abilities. I believe miracles still happen in one way or another to reveal God's presence among us. We also know that miracles rarely happen, and most times it takes the faithful to be convinced.

I believe that most of the time we are given full rights to shape our outcomes in life. My discussion will focus on those who fall into that group—and that's almost all of us.

My job is to help people understand health and how to care for it. We need to do our best to keep ourselves as healthy as we can. We need to understand the role of mutations and genetics in limiting those things that may improve health. These aren't things we can fully control, but doctors will continue to work to help people.

Our discoveries and dedication are gifts from God. Like Jesus Christ told us, seek and you shall find; ask and it will be given to you. The Bible also says that faith without good works is useless. We need to believe and work hard to get the answers to certain things, including what we call paranormal.

We doctors are doing our best to find the answers to the problems we know exist; we don't even know about some problems. I believe there will be more diseases in the future due to ongoing human integration and genetic mutations. Some of the mutations may be from our use of products that may harm our bodies. It could be anything from cigarette smoking, alcohol use, or drug use to different kinds of radiation around us. We could control those harmful products if men and women came together and worked it out. Women, as the ones who carry babies, should understand this. Men should encourage their wives by staying away from those harmful products too, especially in a world where equality in both sexes is misunderstood. The equality is usually with harmful habits, which we can control if we get wiser.

1

Good Health

My health was shaken when I found my blood pressure was in the 140 to 150 systolic range and diastolic range was 95 to 100 especially in the mornings, with a body mass index of twenty-nine. I work in acute care and sometimes have poor sleep habits and an unhealthy lifestyle. I do not smoke or drink, but I was overweight and was not doing any exercise. I saw a change when I stopped drinking juice and started drinking more water and getting more exercise. (Drinking more than 3 liters of water a day can give you the feeling of diuresis, or frequent urnination.) I started playing golf and riding a stationary bicycle, together with getting good sleep. I saw my systolic blood pressure drop from 140 to 119 and my diastolic from 95 to 82 without any medication. I even lost fifteen pounds and had improved sleeping. My snoring has improved markedly, which means I can sleep better and not feel like I am drowning while asleep.

Being overweight or obese could cause sleep apnea and excessive snoring, which means that you are likely *hypoxic*, or have low oxygen. The result is that your body will release adrenaline and other stress hormones as a reaction to the inadequate oxygen supply. That in itself will cause hypertension, with risk of pulmonary hypertension and heart disease. Even though you are sleeping, your body does not get fully rested. This condition is worse when your neck circumference is more than sixteen centimeters. The fat will cause obstruction of your breathing while asleep, which physicians call sleep apnea.

My dad was the youngest of eight siblings. All were very healthy and grew up with good health, but my dad was diabetic. My dad's siblings were educated but not as educated as he was.

He was the only one of the eight with a post-graduate education, and he was the first to die. He went to England as a teenager and later died of complications from diabetes and chronic lung disease. I feel that my dad's family is a typical case study of lifestyle changes and good health.

My dad (may he rest in peace) was a smoker, a habit he picked up in England due to cold weather in an attempt to stay warm. British homes at that time were very poorly insulated and needed a lot of heating to keep them warm. Most of the people in Britain, especially the immigrants, were smokers and tea or coffee drinkers. The lifetime habits of smoking and tea drinking—the tea was with sugar and milk to keep it tasty—resulted in diabetes and chronic lung disease at the age of fifty-three. It became a habit to drink tea instead of water—a habit that is still the norm in the West, especially in England. My dad got used to that lifestyle, as did some of his friends and relations who were there with him. The normal practice of helping his relations in Nigeria resulted in his working more to feed himself and his relations. My dad was obese from those lifestyle changes. He died on December 7, 1999, in the same year that I graduated from medical school. He was a good man.

Other factors could have contributed to his poor health. My dad never explained to his immediate cousins why he'd chosen to marry my mum. There was some misunderstanding about who he should and should not marry. What easily could have been a good thing became misunderstood. It was issue of pride within the family. The misunderstanding continued even when my dad returned to Nigeria with us—my mum, my brother, and me. The cousins involved were first cousins to him and very close. One of them in particular had been special to my dad, as my dad had lived with him while growing up.

My dad had spent so much time in England and had learned so many of the British ways that he was not able initially to understand the issue. It took him some time to understand the tradition at the time. The added stress, together with lifestyle changes, resulted in his early death. He was not only obese and a smoker but a consumer of sugar. I never saw my dad exercise, although he was a very hard worker. All his siblings who did not adopt the lifestyle my dad had lived far longer than he did. Bad habits as well as work stress and uncontrolled obesity led to his early demise.

Yet my dad was the most careful man I have ever met and a very good Christian. I have no doubt he is in heaven. One of my dad's oldest brothers is still alive in his nineties, and he is very healthy and very strong. He also lived in the USA for ten years in the 1990s but lived with his children. He came to the United States after he retired, and he became an American citizen. He's a very good man, and my dad lived most of his early life with him. He taught my dad most of what he knew with regard to social views. He was fifteen years older than my dad and was like a father to him.

Before I talk about obesity and how it could damage our health and lead to other preventable diseases, let me talk about starvation. I will also talk about how having a strong spiritual upbringing can help improve our moods and, at the same time, prevent obesity and make our health better. We live in a world of consumerism and self-interest, which does not help us to make the best choices for our heath. It is a difficult time that may need understanding and God's involvement in our lives. That's my thinking as a person and as a physician.

2

Starvation

Starvation occurs when we have inadequate food intake and poor nutrition. The danger of starvation in the United States or other countries in the developed world is very rare, but it occurs in war-torn areas and parts of Africa, India, and other underdeveloped countries. You see starvation during famines and uncontrolled natural disasters.

The consequences of starvation are poor immunity and poor metabolism. When you have low immunity, you are very predisposed to a lot of infections that may lead to death. Another aspect of poor nutrition is poor muscle development and inflammation, which will lead to heart failure and multiple organ failures. Malnutrition from starvation is also seen in the elderly, especially those who have had bad strokes or have severe dementia. This kind malnutrition is seen all over the world. We use names like "protein calorie malnutrition" or "adult failure to thrive" to describe the condition of some of these people. Usually, most of these patients have refused to eat before becoming malnourished. They usually die from cardiac arrest resulting from the malnutrition.

In the developing world, such as in Africa, we have another form of malnutrition called *kwashiorkor.* It usually results from poor protein intake, and it is very deadly too. It usually is seen in children. The children become very lethargic, with swollen arms and legs. Some have distended abdomens and tiny arms from poor muscle development. Those children, if not fed enough protein, usually die from heart failure. Sometimes they have very slow physical development with poor mental and brain development.

As a medical student and a house officer in Nigeria, I had the opportunity to manage such patients. Sometimes they died from diarrhea and dehydration due to an inability to boost their immunity enough to fight infections when they become ill. Protein products are very expensive in Africa. This results in most mothers feeding their children primarily carbohydrates, which makes them tired and very weak .

Occult malnutrition also occurs in some people due to lack of micronutrients, which can result in poor metabolism and poor development. The symptoms of occult malnutrition may be very vague and difficult to diagnose because they often mimic other illnesses. Some of the micronutrients include vitamins and other nutrients—including zinc, selenium, and cobalt—that are important in helping the body work and function better. They help in building muscles and other parts of the body, even when injured. If those nutrients are not there, the result is the same outcome as starvation, but doctors may be slow to notice the signs. Patients may die if this deficiency is not corrected

During the sixteenth and seventeenth centuries, according to historians like Robert Beverly, there was serious hunger in western Europe that resulted in massive emigration of Europeans to the United States. Starvation and hunger were relatively high in the USA but not compared to Europe or Asia. The life expectancy in the United States was fifty-six years in the seventeenth century, thirty-seven years in Britain, and twenty-eight to thirty years in most parts of Europe.

Due to there being malnutrition in almost every corner of the Western world, countries took it upon themselves to solve the problem. The sixteenth century was also the peak of scientific evolution, which coincided with a strong rise in Christianity in Europe. Faith in Christ was also at the highest point in Christian countries. The result was a big change in solving two of the most important plagues in human history—hunger and starvation.

We have also seen fewer wars, with more countries getting richer. Those rich countries, which we call the developed world, have been able to cure the starvation and hunger problems. For me, that was the biggest achievement in science in human history. However, a new problem arose after that. We went from one extreme to another. The new problem is not as bad as the old one because we live longer, but it is as dangerous. The new problem is obesity and overeating, which we will discuss in the next chapter.

3

Obesity

In the West and all over the world, people are eating more and becoming more sedentary. This is more pronounced in Western countries and is causing more and more obesity. Obesity is a result of overeating and excess calories. The result of such excess eating is that fat is deposited in the wrong places. Those fat deposits can result in poor body function and can prevent proper metabolism. Without proper metabolism, we are at risk for a disease that is now as bad as starvation. Everything taken in excess is bad, and this issue of obesity concludes it. In Africa and some parts of Asia, most obese people die from what local people call "the rich-man disease." Currently, almost every one of those countries is affected, but obesity is still more prevalent in the ones with exposure to Western culture; that is, those with enough finances to buy whatever they want. The common diseases involved include coronary artery disease, which is basically plaque in the blood vessels supplying the heart. There is also a high incidence of stroke, congestive heart failure, and hypertension.

In the West, the opposite is becoming the case, as more rich people tend to improve on their lifestyles and diets compared to others. Still, obesity is present across all ethnic groups and social classes in the USA.

A sedentary lifestyle is an important cause of obesity in the West, especially in the United States. In most states, in both urban and rural areas, most people drive to work or to grocery stores. The weather conditions and location of grocery stores have made it inevitable that people will drive.

A sedentary lifestyle is one in which we take fewer than five thousand steps a day; we see this across the board in the United States. The industrialization of the world resulted in massive food production. The availability of machines made it possible for us to work less and produce more. It helped in taking care of food shortages, but at the same time, it affected our way of life.

I would like to address calorie intake. When we take in more calories than we use, we store the excess calories as fat, which results in weight gain. Soda industries make soda available to the public, which results in addiction to their products. They are also creating jobs as well, making a good and bad thing. We have sugary products in different forms, including chocolates, juice, candy, and ice cream. Those companies create jobs and help to decrease unemployment in the country.

Eating and drinking sugary beverages is not bad if done in moderation. Obesity is defined by a body mass index of more than thirty. A lot of the public are in this category. Obesity becomes *morbid obesity* when the body mass index is more than forty. The consequences of obesity are quite extensive. The job of health care workers is to prevent obesity and improve people's lives. One of the ways to prevent obesity is to check our weight, and see if we can keep our body mass index at twenty to twenty-five. For men, twenty-six or twenty-seven may not be a bad idea, especially for a black person who may have a higher muscle density. The body mass index is calculated by dividing your weight in kilograms by your height in meters squared (kg/m^2).

If you are in that obese range, the best way to cut your weight is to stop drinking any sugary product. That will be enough to reduce the weight to the required level. If you are someone who does not drink any sugar, then you have to cut down on your meals. You can do that by maybe halving your lunch to get the appropriate result.

Our family experience has shown me that any kind of excess sugar consumption is bad for the body.

What constitutes good health?

Good health is seen when we eat and exercise in a way that keeps our weight in the required range. Most people are less active as they get older, especially in their thirties and forties. This means that our tendency toward obesity may increase with age. The consequences may include accelerated aging and early onset hypertension.

Hypertension can be very damaging to the body by causing various diseases, including heart disease, stroke, and renal failure. Normal blood pressure in the average person is 120/80, and we usually perfuse or supply blood to our body's internal organs very well at a pressure of 90/60. When we become heavier than normal, however, we tend to put more pressure on our heart to do more. This is possibly because our bodies need to adjust our blood pressure to perfuse our larger mass. Those changes will lead to the consequences listed above.

Obese people are also more likely to have problems with sleep, which will result in sleep apnea. Sleep apnea is a moment of not breathing while asleep. During those times, our oxygen is lower, and that low oxygen will negatively affect our bodies' blood pressure. Low oxygen likely will increase the stress hormones in the body, which also force the body's blood pressure to increase, leading to hypertension. High blood pressure will result in micro-injury to the blood vessels, and this can cause damage to the organs. Also with obesity, the fats can cause higher cholesterol than usual, which can be another factor that causes more problems to internal organs, including atherosclerotic disease, which is usually a weak vessel as compared to normal ones.

Because those vessels are weak, there is a strong risk of stroke and heart disease, including heart attack and heart failure, atrial fibrillation, and other arrhythmias, which can cause clots in the heart that may result in stroke. Obesity and fat deposits in the wrong places also may lead to fat in the spleen and bones and other organs, which will prevent these organs from working the way they should.

Obese people tend to develop infections very easily, as the body's immunity is affected by abnormal fat in the bones and other organs, thus preventing them from functioning optimally. The pancreas also is affected by abnormal fat deposits, resulting in poor sugar metabolism, which leads to diabetes mellitus. Insulin resistance is also noted, as the insulin receptors do not function properly. The heart also functions poorly, with initial diastolic failure and increased work for the heart.

Another big problem is arthritis and joint pain, as the body is carrying more weight than it can handle. The first joint to be affected is usually the knees and then the hip or back. Body function works optimally when the body mass index is less than twenty-six.

Currently in the United States, one of the most common causes of disease in young people is obesity due to overeating and unnecessary excess calorie intake.

I helped rehabilitate multiple cases of obesity. One of my patients, however, died from a heart attack six months after discharge from the rehab center. During rehabilitation, he lost 150 pounds and dropped from 550 pounds to 400, which was a sizeable chunk. He went home and then relapsed and started eating a lot of calories and junk again. He regained one hundred pounds afterward.

My initial intention was to keep him in the rehab center for at least a year to avoid relapse. Due to logistics, however, and the fact he preferred being home to being in a nursing home, he was discharged early—no one can keep a person against his own wishes. Prior to coming to the nursing home, he had developed a bad heart from severe obesity, and our job was to give him a chance. He had a defibrillator with his heart pumping at 25 percent of normal. He could have improved if he had agreed on the lifestyle changes we tried to instill in him.

We were proud of a patient who was a pastor. He was put on hospice because of recurrent hospital admission due to complications of obesity. He already had significant heart disease and difficult-to-control diabetes. He was in his early sixties, which is usually the expected life span of the morbidly obese, especially those with complications. While on hospice, he decided to go to the hospital for treatment after he developed a very bad infection in his lungs. He was treated and then decided to have rehabilitation in the nursing home. While there, he had his weight checked every three days, and he lost one hundred pounds, bringing his weight down to 350 pounds. To his surprise, his congestive heart failure also improved, and his diabetes was better controlled. He also noted that his susceptibility to leg infections had improved. He stayed with me for six months and lost another thirty pounds and was able to walk with a cane. As of this writing, he uses two canes to walk; previously, he could not walk at all.

He went home, and I followed his progress for another three months to prevent relapse. He did very well—he is out of hospice and has not been admitted to the hospital in the last two years.

A major problem that is very common with

obesity, especially morbid obesity, is a leg infection called cellulitis. We had a patient who came to the hospital almost every three to six months with cellulitis. She has refused rehabilitation in the nursing home. I think the insurance company and Medicare should encourage such people to do rehab because it is putting too much pressure on tax money to keep morbidly obese people out of the hospital. Rehabilitation should be the key in combating chronic diseases. The nurses and the rehabilitation specialists are also a big plus on this adventure.

Obese patients may develop infections that sometimes get into their blood, causing sepsis from the cellulitis. This also could be avoided by rehabilitating to lose fifty to one hundred pounds. Usually, we treat them with intravenous antibiotics for two to three weeks to get the infection out of their systems. Average-weight people can easily be treated with oral antibiotics most of the time. The morbidly obese are difficult to treat, especially if they have diabetes complicating their situations. The worst part is that some of them get very angry when we tell them the origin of their problem. That's where I think spiritual help may help in communicating the problem.

It is also good to highlight to them how difficult it is to treat them because of how big they are. If they go into respiratory failure, it is usually difficult to get them intubated. The nurses also have to change and turn them once in a while, and that can be very difficult. Most of them cannot turn by themselves. At the age of fifty to sixty years they are finding it difficult to stand from a seated position. They usually need help with almost everything. They often become very disabled, meaning they are now sedentary and will need to depend mostly on dieting and rehab specialists to put them back to normal

The issue with cellulitis in these patients can be a challenge to doctors because the infection usually affects both legs, and they often have other medical problems, like diabetes, congestive heart failure, and difficulty breathing. They are difficult to examine because the stethoscope may not notice any sound when the abdomen is big and distended.

The other sad part is trying to take images that will help in making a diagnosis. Some of these people cannot fit into an MRI or CT scan to get tested. Some of them even don't x-ray properly—it often will show many dense shadows, and it's almost impossible to make any sense of it. We have to rely on the patient's medical history to make a sense of what they have. It's a specialized skill to treat obese people. I will not advise them to be managed by just any health care worker; they need an experienced qualified physician. The mortality rate of these patients in the hospital is very high, and that is why it is a matter of urgency to treat them.

4

Diet

In the United States of America, food is readily available to the public. The government provides welfare to the poor in order to help alleviate poverty. Those are very good measures to prevent starvation, especially in most rich countries. The country is also doing well economically, which means there is food for the masses. The problem is overeating and not eating the right foods. A good diet consists of about two thousand calories a day, especially for someone who is somewhat active. It may be difficult to calculate calories, but the best way is to check your weight regularly, and if you gain weight, then cut out the ice cream, chocolate, potato chips etc... you are eating. If you like sugary bread, such as you see in Dunkin' Donuts, maybe it is time to pass on that. My observations have told me that it is not easy to gain weight if your source of fluid is just water and not sugary soda. If a 150-pound man eats three meals a day and drinks two cups of soda once a week, it will be difficult to become obese. The obesity comes from snacking and drinking soda. It also is difficult to gain weight if you drink a bottle of beer or a glass of wine once a week.

Adding vegetables to our meals will help to improve digestion and help us to feel full. Eating light toast at breakfast and then a good lunch with some vegetables and one liter of water will help us enjoy our food. Drinking about three liters of water a day not only helps you to eat the right amount of food but will help get rid of salt. The urine always has salt but water has no salt. Water also acts as a diuretic and therefore is very good for blood pressure control.

The diet should include fruits, which have a lot of electrolytes and will help to make the stomach feel full. Fruits also provide potassium and other micronutrients that will prevent occult malnutrition and low blood pressure. Fruit is natural and not processed.

Some people have a food addiction and an inability to drink water. Food addiction can be helped with rehabilitation—we help the person to think less about food during rehab. Depression may be a significant part of overeating, but using my experience from Africa and England, where foods are not as available as in the USA, I know that it is possible to rehabilitate these people if the family understands the problem early and tells the doctor about it. Food addiction usually starts very early, before high school, and continues until it becomes a big problem.

My own problem with obesity (which I solved by myself after I developed hypertension and sleep apnea) started in England. My hypertension started because I was drinking a lot of juice instead of water. Juice was my source of fluid, and I gained weight, jumping from 143 pounds to 187 pounds in less than ten years. I just had to stop the juice, and that on its own dropped my weight significantly. Now I eat my usual quantity of food and drink 2.5 liters of water every day, which also helped in getting me to eat less. My blood pressure dropped from 145/100 to 119/79. My current body mass index is 26.5, and my target is 25 or 26, which I think is good for me.

There are many books about antioxidants, which our bodies need. The fruits that provide most of the available nutrients include bananas, oranges, mango, guava, strawberries, and grapes. Eating one or two of those fruits each day should be okay, especially at lunchtime. The problem in the USA is that some of those fruits are barely ripe before they are sold to the community, or some are spoiled before the consumer gets them. The result is that they taste acidic, and people are discouraged from eating them.

Salad with broccoli and carrots, in addition to your food and fruits, should make a good lunch, and those should be enough for the day.

At night, you can eat what you like but no soda—just water as suggested. Try to eat a cup and a half of food for supper to allow you to sleep well at night. Sleeping is very important, as we will discuss in another chapter. Having a nice meal and a good sleep—one is as good as the other.

I also encourage people to add a multivitamin to their diets. Maintaining an optimal weight and eating a balanced diet with no weight gain will keep you from getting infections and inflammations that will result in poor health. Poor health may prevent you from exercising the way you should. Good health encourages us to work at our most optimal level. I encourage families to use multivitamins with vitamin D and selenium. Selenium is known to help in fighting viral infection. It actually has been shown to help reduce the effect of HIV on the body. HIV is a virus, and selenium has been shown to play a good part in controlling viruses. Viral infection can prevent us from engaging in our normal exercise routine or eating a balanced diet. When we are sick we tend not to eat well or drink enough water. We tend to like high carbohydrate foods such as noodles or pasta and foods that may affect our ability to care for our health. I also think that viral infection may affect our moods and induce other autoimmune diseases. Those autoimmune diseases may affect our moods and also jeopardize our plan to effectively accomplish our goal. Staying away from viral infection will help to prevent inflammation and also will improve our work ethic.

Winter weather often forces most people to stay indoors, but staying indoors can affect our ability to make enough vitamin D in our system. Vitamin D has been is an immune modulator and is helpful in our day-to-day activity. It is a very important vitamin in calcium and magnesium metabolism and also in phosphorus metabolism. Phosphorous is one of the electrolytes that helps the body with energy. It is a product of ATP, which is the chemical by which our bodies store energy. Vitamin D research has been extensive, as most people with diabetes have responded well to it. We may think we can keep healthy with vitamin D, but all vitamins are good, and our bodies need them to function properly and to prevent infections and heart disease.

5

Exercise and Health

Exercise is one of the best ways of keeping good health. The best exercise is to exercise in what you love to do. In that way, you don't feel stressed about it. You don't need to go through the pressure of work and then come home again to feel the pressure from exercise. Exercise should be relaxing, with a feel-good attitude to it. Enjoying exercise definitely will help you to improve your health.

During exercise, our blood vessels dilate, which is why we sweat. Perspiration cool our bodies when they warm up from exercise. The increase in blood flow to the skin usually helps in the process of sweat to cool the body. Exercise also causes an increased blood flow to the other organs, resulting in increased metabolism in those organs, especially the muscles. The increase in metabolism will result in the production of energy, which helps our bodies to function better. It also helps us burn calories

One of the problems I've seen is people trying to exercise like professional athletes at the age of forty. This causes unnecessary exhaustion to the body, making it counterproductive. Even professional athletes are encouraged to retire, not just because they are getting tired but because they would harm themselves if they continued to train at that level. The health risk of excessive training at a certain age is high and includes arthritis and other injuries to the body. My goal in teaching people about exercise is to help them build up their endurance. Start slow and gradually increase the length of exercise until you reach a point of comfort. The best exercise is the exercise that gets you to break some sweat a couple of times a day.

In summary, exercising at a later stage in life

to stay healthy should be done in moderation. I've seen people who hire trainers and coaches to help them with exercise. These often poorly trained coaches sometimes subject their clients to serious muscle injury and exhaustion. It's a kind of surgical approach to exercise. They want their client to lose ten pounds in one day. This book will help trainers and trainees know what to expect and how to go about it. My guide here will probably help these trainers to be more considerate in getting their clients to the appropriate weight slowly, instead of in a day or in a week.

I also know some patients who have started an exercise program themselves to get to the appropriate weight, and they get themselves in so much trouble that some of them end up in the ICU.

A lot of professional athletes are on a particular diet to help avoid some of the injuries I've mentioned. Their bodies are conditioned to such exercises, and I will tell you how that is possible. One of the problems with severe exercise is muscle ache and pain after exercise. Those pains may be so intense that the athlete ends up in the emergency room because the muscle ache and pain is unbearable.

A case in point is a thirty-year-old man who I managed as a resident physician, with the help of the nephrologist and the critical care physician in New York. The young man, who was very fit and looked athletic, wanted to have a six pack in his abdomen, so he went into the gym to make his dreams come true. He was in the gym for two hours building his biceps and abdominal walls. He wanted to achieve those objectives in one day. He had not exercised for almost two years now but wanted a surgical approach to building his muscles. He also did some treadmill and some heavy lifting. On coming home, he slept and then woke up with muscle ache and soreness. When he arrived at the emergency room, his blood draw revealed a high level of a chemical called CPK, or creatine phosphate kinase. This chemical is present in the body normally because we continuously use our muscles. The normal level is less than 400 in almost everyone. The level goes up when we have muscle ache, either from a fall, a virus infection, or any injury to the muscle.

This young man had a CPK level of more than 35,000, which resulted in admission to the intensive care unit. It was a wise decision to come to the hospital, as he was then started on intravenous fluid to prevent his kidneys from shutting down. At a very high level, CPK can cause a kidney shut-down by blocking the small tubules in the kidney. He needed a lot of fluid intravenously to prevent this.

People thus affected can be in the hospital from a day up to two weeks—we keep them until the physician is comfortable with discharging them. The usual level that tends to harm a patient is around 2,000. Patients are usually discharged after the CPK is down, and they are encouraged to drink a lot of water.

Muscle breakdown also includes an increase in uric acid and high potassium, which can cause a heart attack. The increase in potassium is because potassium is present in the muscle cell, which when injured from the intensive exercise will result in an increased level. The high level may result in heart arrhythmia and possibly death, if very severe.

The most important problem is that sometimes the muscle swelling may continue to release the chemical, and then we may need a special dialysis in a tertiary hospital. We usually keep patients until they are safe. If the condition does not improve after a day or two, we encourage them to be transferred to a tertiary hospital, where they have other specialists.

If the heart muscle is put under the same pressure, it may result in heart attack, especially if the heart is already weak or compromised. I have seen patients die suddenly after exercise, and some develop significant heart disease, requiring intensive care on life support.

One reasons for muscle breakdown is lactic acid, which is usually produced when we have poor blood circulation or serious infections. Normally, when we have excess muscle activity, we may injure ourselves this way. Our muscle energy normally is produced from glucose metabolism during exercise. Some of the glucose will convert to lactic acid to produce additional energy. Some of these lactic acids, if not well metabolized, will cause muscle injury at the cell level and may lead to muscle swelling and soreness.

To prevent muscle injury, we try to encourage people to exercise gradually and build up mitochondria in the cells. The mitochondria is that part of the cell where energy is produced at the molecular level. When we exercise for fifteen minutes daily and then increase to twenty minutes daily the next week and then thirty minutes daily the next month, we gradually increase the mitochondria density. Increasing the mitochondria density is very important to help metabolize any lactic acid, which will cause some of these muscle injuries in our heart muscles or body muscle. In that way, we condition our bodies and then prevent muscle soreness and injury.

We need to gradually increase the mitochondria numbers (density) in the muscle to help prevent injury and soreness from lactic acid. The heart muscle will adapt as well to handle more activity during exercise.

By increasing our metabolism and burning calories, we tend to lose weight.

Excess calories cause an increase in weight, especially when we take more than what our body needs. When we exercise to increase metabolism, we also allow insulin to work better, which allows more glucose into the muscle to be metabolized to produce energy. The muscle, which functions better because of less fat around the receptors, will prevent insulin resistance and diabetes mellitus. Some people have seen their diabetes improved after lifestyle changes and exercise.

Remember that the definition of a sedentary lifestyle is fewer than five thousand steps a day. The required steps a day to prevent obesity and maintain good health is six thousand to ten thousand steps a day. The average required calories per day is 1,800 to 2,400, depending on your height and level of activity. It's important not to be sedentary because our bodies have naturally evolved to function actively and move. If we don't move, our joints may stiffen and our muscles may become small.

The immune functions improve with exercise, as more blood flow to the organs will help improve immunity. With an increase in exercise and blood flow, the blood vessel dilatation helps in normalizing blood pressure. Hypertension will be prevented as heart muscle and resting heart rate is improved. Hypertension, in the long run, is improved with exercise, due to our bodies' structural changes. Those structural changes help to prevent hypertension.

My brand of exercise is golf, running, and sometimes lawn tennis to break a sweat. I try to play in a par-three nine-hole course without a golf cart. I have been able to decrease my blood pressure with those light exercises.

I try to exercise at least three times a week and then walk about six thousand steps the rest of the week. I have also seen an improvement in my breathing and a decrease in snoring. I wake up strong instead of feeling tired. My diet and exercise program started about three months ago, and the changes I have noted are remarkable. I have talked to patients to help guide them in their lifestyle changes. Lifestyle change is difficult but attainable. It requires our will and some spiritual guidance. The spiritual guidance is usually through our effort. When we have those two, we can move any mountain in front of us. The problem today is that, unlike in the sixteenth century when Christianity was rising, it now is fading gradually. Science originated from Christian countries after they found purpose in Christ. That purpose resulted in fulfilling Christ's promise of "ask and we shall find" and "seek and it will be given to us." We used that purpose to solve starvation and understand other parts of our world. also known as the universe. We were able to acquire knowledge and transfer the knowledge to our peers so they could improve on it. However, great scientists, like Isaac Newton, who were strong spiritual men likely would weep (if they were still alive), as science is turning us against God instead of turning us to God. We acquired knowledge and improved on our well-being, and then we became complacent and irresponsible. We have seen in the last decade that the life expectancy is falling instead of rising. More people per capita died this year than two or three years ago. More young people are hooked on drugs, alcohol, and bad health care activities than we have ever seen. The repercussions of turning away from spiritual guidance is worsening by day, and data out there confirms it. Before we talk more on spirituality and health, I'll elaborate on the importance of sleep.

6

Sleeping and Health

Sleeping is one of the most important factors in keeping good health. When you sleep, you allow your body to heal and also allow your brain to reset. I recommend at least seven hours of sleep to be able to have good judgment when awake. When we sleep at night, we go through fasting for twelve hours. During sleep, our bodies are quiet to allow the body to heal. Most of our natural hormones increase at night during sleep. Those hormones help with healing of the injured muscles. This includes the growth hormones that are known to help with metabolism and healing of injured cells.

Problems with poor sleep include hypertension

and recurrent brain activity and tiredness. Another common problem with poor sleep is muscle pain and micro-injuries of the muscles and bones, which will not heal very well. Muscle soreness and pains may result in depression if not handled well.

One of the most common problems of CEOs, doctors, and some professionals is poor sleep. They are doing well with exercise, yet a significant number of them become depressed due to stress. About four hundred doctors in the USA commit suicide every year from stress and depression. I saw a CEO who was looking very fit and who exercised very well, but he slept less than four hours a day. This CEO later died from a heart attack at the age of forty-three. He did everything right for his health—except he was sleeping very poorly. The result of poor sleep is increased inflammatory markers in the body, which may result in coronary artery disease and hypertension. With poor sleep, we have an increase in cathecolamines in the body, which may cause hypertension and increase the resting heart rate. The person may easily develop coronary artery disease and die from heart attack. There is also an increase in the cortisol level, which is very bad when it is at higher than normal levels. Cortisol is a steroid hormone, and like most steroids, when they are not working the way they should, they tend to increase the risk of hypertension and diabetes.

There are two main cycles in sleep: rapid eye movement (REM) and non-rapid eye movement (NREM). They are responsible for the cycles of deep sleep and light sleep and also dreams. Those cycles are very important to good health. As mentioned, we need seven hours of sleep to fulfill those important cycles and maintain good health. Excessive use of stimulants, such as caffeine, tends to affect our sleep. Pressure at work also messes up our sleep patterns. The anxiety of waking up early and drinking coffee to keep awake could be a major problem to our health. When you are anxious about waking up early, you may end up not sleeping at all. When you don't sleep well, you put yourself in a difficult condition. Waking in the night or waking too early is akin to torture when it comes to our health care. We also run another risk by drinking stimulants to keep awake. These lifestyle choices will harm our bodies severely in the long and short run. They may increase our chances of coronary artery disease and hypertension, which will also lead to significant heart disease, diabetes, stroke, and death.

7

The Spiritual Role

Meditation and spiritual richness help to achieve our goals. When we have spiritual richness, we have something to look up to.

After learning of my dad's story about his mum's apparition, I have no doubt about an afterlife and that God works in ways we don't know.

It is impossible to use our minds to understand God the way we would like to. We see the changes that occur in the world, and though we may attribute them to our ingenuity, there is more to it. It is important that we understand that God plays a part in our lives, though it may not be fully defined, like one plus one equals two. A lack of this knowledge of God may affect our ability to live a healthy life and achieve our goals.

We can control our health with our own will, but it may be very challenging if we have no God in our lives. It is not easy to *not* to believe in God. It may look easy, but it is tormenting if the world around us becomes blurry and incomprehensible. People with poor will power, not due to a fault of their own making, seek help with disturbing lifestyle changes. Those lifestyle changes may be harmful to them and to the people who care for them. They may partially have the will to be spiritually strong but not the will to be spiritually active.

It may be easy to live life as if there is no tomorrow, but in the end, people who love you will cry if trouble arises from such a lifestyle. Living for those people is a kind of spiritual riches, as you understand life as something related to you. You understand that you are not alone in this world. You understand that people love you. You understand the downside of selfishness.

In my opinion, we should try to merge a positive attitude with strong spiritual knowledge to achieve an optimum lifestyle that will impact people around us in a positive way. That attitude will help us to put more effort in caring for ourselves, attempting to live a healthy life, and looking to help people related to us. It also frees our minds from personal preventable torture, which is the real freedom we crave.

I have witnessed some of my patients' stories of the afterlife after they were resuscitated from death. Some of their stories did not have a strong scientific proof, but the conviction in their stories is worthy of notice. It could be a result of brain interpretation of the event at the time, but the stories are very remarkable. I had a patient who, after resuscitation, refused to talk to me because she was sure she had been in a beautiful place full of flowers and a beautiful garden. She said she could not describe it by mouth, but she did not want to leave. She said, "Do not resuscitate me again!" She was quick to tell her family that they should not miss her when she died again. She was in her nineties with myocardial infarction. Her conviction of the event was remarkable.

Important scientists such as Galileo Galilei (1564–1643; rest in peace) did remarkable work as Christians to help in bringing us to the level of world understanding today. I will also give special credit to Robert Boyle (1791–1867; rest in peace) who did great work on gases, known as Boyle's law. Boyle wrote a book showing that his studies in science were strictly based on his Christian belief. He basically said that understanding Christ was the fundamental of science. He published a lot of books and paid money to help preach Christianity outside Christian faith.

Copernicus, a Polish man and also a canon in Catholic Church, published a mathematical formula to describe the rotation of planets around the sun. His work was scrutinized, and he was quick to point out that the knowledge of Christ and the Bible led him to the research and publication. Today's world will not tell you about the faith of those respectable scientists of the fourteenth to the twentieth centuries— scientists who did tremendous work out of their faith in Christianity. Their names are numerous, including Michael Faraday, Francis Bacon, Rene Descartes, Jacques Charles (Charles's law), and our twentieth-century genius Albert Einstein, who was not an outspoken faith member but did not hide his belief in God as the Creator of universe. His conviction was based on the work put by those special men mentioned above, who made it possible for a Jewish man to understand science as he did. Their belief was rooted on Christianity and faith, which I sometimes interpret as hard work with strong conviction, based on your belief that Christ and the Bible was right. With such guidance and belief, those scientists changed the world and made it a better place. They also proved themselves right by showing that Christ was right in his teachings.

Today's science is changing and current teachings are contrary to that of the original founders. Scientists preach a more and more godless world, with expanding laziness in their work. The groundbreaking scientific world of the fourteenth to eighteenth centuries seems more interesting than today's scientific world, which sometimes is full of hit-or-miss observations without strong guidance.

Those changes are a result of distorted minds, which have weakened us. The mind is a strong indication of the body, not just a mass or matter that is worth nothing but dust. Sir Francis Bacon's speech on the mind and God being interlocked in philosophy needs attention.

We need those of strong will to understand what our health means to us and how to keep it healthy, not just for ourselves but for our children, families, and friends. We are not alone in this world, and we need to know that. I believe that if we can understand that little theory, we will have started a journey of spiritual fullness filled with love and kindness.

About the Author

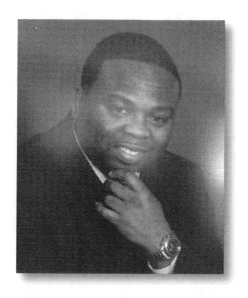

David Ilo was born to Mathias and Grace Ilo in Birmingham, England. His siblings are Joel Chuka Ilo, a pharmacist in Texas; Judith Okonkwo; Winifred, Euphemia, and Lidia Ilo; and the late Esther Ilo (rest in peace).

He started school in Nigeria and later attended high school at the College of Immaculate

Conception in Enugu, Nigeria, and university at the University of Nigeria, Nsukka and Enugu campuses. He did his residency at St. John's Episcopal Hospital in Far Rockaway, New York, a division of State University of New York (SUNY). He graduated from medical school in 2000.

Dr. Ilo is a British citizen by birth, a Nigerian citizen by parental origin, and a naturalized US citizen. Apogee Physicians (the largest entirely physician-owned and operated hospitalist group in the nation) sponsored his green card.

He has published work on stem cells and is a board-certified physician in the United States. He currently works with geriatric and hospice groups as well as working in acute care as a hospitalist in Indiana. He loves his job and helping patients.

Dr. Ilo is married to the former Piper Smith.